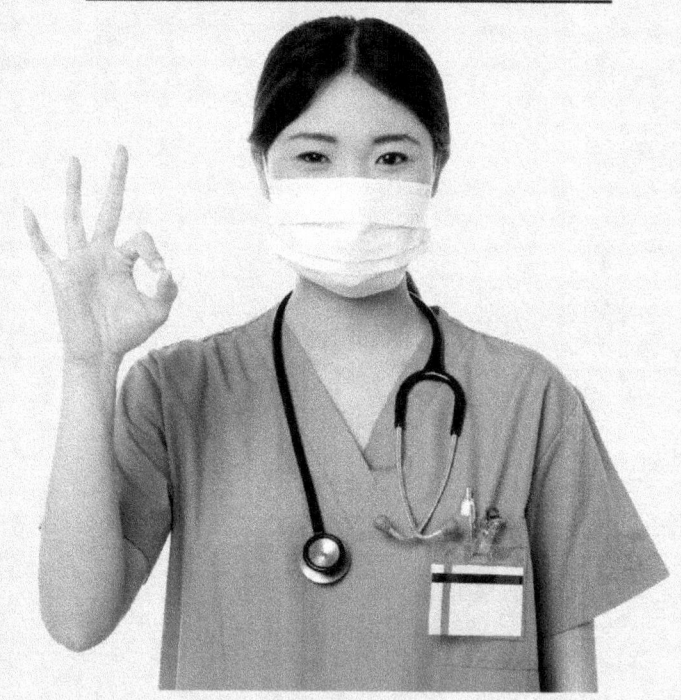

HEALTH CARE ETHICS FOR NURSES

Magna Anissa Edding Aming-Hayudini, RN, RM, LPT, MAN, MPA, DPA

1st Edition

HEALTH CARE ETHICS
For Nurses
1st Edition

Copyright @2021 by
Magna Anissa Edding Aming-Hayudini

ISBN 978-1-105-77141-5
Published by Lulu Book Publishing

United States of America

Foreword

This book is intended for medical practitioners, specifically nurses. The author's desire to simplify the Health Care Ethics in nursing practice will help readers embrace its significance.

However, the legal concerns and issues are discussed in this book to educate beginning nurses in academe and the practice setting. It may also guide nurses to become more competent in caring for patients as possible.

The author believes that this first book will provide a light understanding of ethical principles in healthcare settings.

Magna Anissa Edding Aming-Hayudini,
RN,RM,LPT,MAN,MPA,DPA-

DEDICATION

This book is heartily dedicated to my family, especially my loving husband, Al-widar Hayudini, and my son Al-Nizhar.

It is also dedicated to my beloved parents, Hji. Magsaysay Aming and Hja Nasura Edding-Aming and Hja. Tindah Halipa-Hayudini, my supportive siblings, namely: Dr. Arsheema A. Abdurahman and Dr. Jonrad Abdurahman, Hja. Mardhia A. Kulod and P/C Abdulbasit Kulod, JD Safia Edding Aming, Dr. Rofaida Edding Aming, Hja. Shehada A. Alih and Saide M. Alih, Hja. Brenda A. Hussin and Emerkhan Hussin, and Hja. Nurmina Aming.

Lastly, this book is dedicated to the Graduate School, Mindanao State University-Sulu, Patikul, Sulu.

Magna Anissa Edding Aming-Hayudini

CONTENTS

Chapter 1

Introduction to Ethics

What is Ethics – It is the science relating to moral actions and moral values. According to Boyer et al., 1991, "Ethics encompasses principles of right or good conduct or a body of such principles."

Ethical Theories

a. **Normative Theories** – are universally applicable, involve questions and dilemmas requiring a choice of action, and entail a conflict of rights and obligations on the nurse/decision-maker.

b. **Deontological Theories** – It derives norms and rules from the duties human beings owe one another under commitments made and roles assumed.

   1. **Situation Ethics** – the decision-making considers the unique characteristics of each individual, the caring relationship between the person and the caregiver, and the most

humanistic course of action given the circumstances.

2. **Act Deontology** – is based on the personal moral values of the person making the ethical situation.

3. **Rule Deontology** – is based on the belief that specific ethical decisions transcend the individual's moral values.

c. **Teleological Theories** – derive norms or rules for conduct from the consequences of actions. Right consists of beneficial consequences, and bad consists of destructive consequences.

d. **Utilitarianism** – makes an action right or wrong is its utility with beneficial actions bringing out the greatest good for the greatest number of people.[1]

1. **Rule Utilitarianism** – seeks the greatest happiness for all. It appeals to the public agreement as a basis for objective judgment about the nature of happiness.

2. **Act Utilitarianism** – attempts to determine which course of action will bring about the greatest happiness or the least harm and suffering that makes happiness subjective.

e. **Principalism** – incorporates various existing ethical principles and attempts to resolve conflicts by applying one or more principles. It controls professional decision-making much more in ethical concerns.

Guide to Maintain Legal Rights within Ethical Dilemmas:

- Recognize the difference between legal rights and ethical views.
- Nurses must realize that their ethical views and values may differ significantly from the patient's value system.
- Nurses must remain current about the recent judicial decisions in their jurisdiction and incorporate these standards and rights into nursing care.
- Nurses are recommended to remove themselves from patients' nursing care if values come into a major conflict. Example: If the mechanical ventilator supports a terminally ill person to live because their family doesn't want the patient to die.
- Ethical Dilemmas have no perfect answers, just a better answer.[1]

Ethical Principles

Autonomy – addresses personal freedom and self-determination. The right to choose what will happen to one's person. Example: The legal doctrine of informed consent.

Beneficence – states that the actions one takes should promote good action.

Nonmaleficence – states the one shall not harm. Example: Do not stress patients during their admission.

Veracity – It concerns truth-telling and incorporates the concept that individuals should always tell the truth.

Fidelity – It is keeping one's promises or commitments. Example: If one is a victim of crime, never divulge to anyone.

Paternalism – It is also known as paternalism that allows one to make decisions for another and is often seen as an undesirable principle. It is the standards of best interest that will help the patient decide on her health care.

Justice – states that people should be treated fairly and equally.

Respect for others – It is the highest form of treatment. It is to acknowledge individuals' right to make decisions and live or die with this decision.[2]

Chapter 2
Health Care Ethics

The course aims to develop in students an understanding of the important concepts and principles of Bioethics. At the end of the course, students should be sensitive to ethical considerations and face ethical issues in patient care, community work, and public issues responsibly.

It applies the core principles of bioethics, law, medical and health care decisions, and responsibilities.[1,2]

Fundamentals of Philosophy and Bioethics

Rationale: Every aspect of medical practice is governed by sets of ethical standards that are to be followed. Therefore, the content of this lesson will give them a perspective on how philosophy affects the action and decision making and capability of the students in any setting.

Nature of Philosophy:

Philosophy --------------------> Thinking

*The act of questioning or wanting to know initiates philosophy and relates philosophy to thinking most of the time.[3]

***Philosophy** - comes from 2 Greek words; **Philos - Love and Sophia - Knowledge/Wisdom**. It is defined as the knowledge of all things through ultimate cause and acquired through reasoning. Its main objective is to seek the most profound explanation of existence and the nature of being. It explicitly uses logic to show its natural scope in deriving those explanations.

***Love of Wisdom** - to the task that requires a deliberate effort to seek the truth.

***Philosopher** - lover of knowledge; a person who seeks knowledge for its own sake and not for any other motive.[3]

Brief History Of Philosophy

Philosophy started at the age of western civilization. It took place in Athens in the 5th Century

***Ancient/Pre-Socratic (7th Century B.C.)** - Greek thinkers called themselves "wise men" but out of humility. **Pythagoras**, one of the Greek thinkers, wanted to call himself a person who just loves wisdom or a "Philosopher."[4]

***Medieval/Middle Ages** - Christian scholars and Arab philosophers were the first philosophers who directly linked philosophy to theology, one of its main inspirations in the Christian faith, which became a stimulus to reason.

*Modern (17th – 18th Century A.D.) – Rene Descartes was known as the father of Modern Philosophy, to his philosophy of rationalism and empiricism. **Rationalism** is a philosophical doctrine that specifies the uses of reasoning and proof in explaining reality. **Empiricism** regards experience as the only source of knowledge.

*Contemporary (20th Century) – the existence of a great variety of doctrines of a philosophy strengthened its grasp in seeking the truth. Among these are the doctrines of **Marxism by Karl Marx, Kantianism by Immanuel Kant,** and **Existentialism by Jean-Paul Sarte.**[4]

Philosophy And The Nature Of Man

1. As a living organism – feeding himself for nutrition, growing and reproducing to preserve his race.

2. As organism to senses – acquires sensory knowledge through; External and Internal Senses

   External – smell, taste and touch(nutrition), hearing and sight (cognition)

   Internal – consciousness, imagination, memory, and instincts

3. As an organism to senses, man tends to be aware of good things through his emotions.
4. As a rational organism to senses, man acquires knowledge by using his free will in judging and reasoning.
5. As an intellectual organism, man uses his conscience to make a practical judgment in choosing a good from an evil action.[5]

The Concept Of Professional Ethics And Bioethics

*It began to be discussed in the 1960s when such phrases as "medical ethics" and "biomedical ethics" were in fashion. The term was originally from America. **Van Reusselaer Potter**, a cancer researcher, claims to have invented the word in a book entitled 'Bioethics: Bridge to the Future.'

Ethics – Greek (Ethos) – Characteristics way of acting; Latin (Mos, Morrs) – way of acting.

 *It is the study of human acts or conducts from a moral perspective as to whether they are good or bad. It is associated with customs, morals, and etiquette and even used interchangeably.

Customs – are acts approved by a group or society.

Etiquette – social observance required by good breeding

Parts of Ethics

1. General Ethics – deals with the basic principles in the life of a man as a member of society.
2. Social Ethics – tackles the basic principles in a man's life as a member of society.

Objectives of Ethics

1. To live an orderly social life
2. To make clear to us why one act is better than the other.
3. To appraise and criticize the moral conduct and ethical system intelligently
4. To seek the true value of life.[5]

Chapter 3
Bioethics

Professional Ethics – It is a branch of moral science that treats the obligations that a member of a profession owes to the public, his profession, and his clients.

*Bioethics – Bio + Ethics = Life

Bioethics – is the term used to describe the application of ethics to biological sciences, medicine, and related fields. It is a systematic study of moral conduct in life sciences and medicines. Thus, a special focus on challenges arising from modern biotechnology is applied.[1]

Scope of Bioethics

1. Concerned with ethical problems associated with medical practices and biosciences
2. The problem of bioethics has something to do with the challenges posed by the biotechnological advances and their power over life and death.

3. Deal with the questions about human life in 3 different points.

   *The beginning of life (contraception and family planning)

   * Amid life (Genetic Engineering and Abortion)

   *At the end of life (Death Penalty and Euthanasia)

Importance or Significance of Bioethics:

1. To provide awareness to the health team or workers of the "dos and "don'ts" medical practice.
2. To enrich one's competence by understanding that a patient is a person and holistic individual

(Ethics employs the marvelous faculty of human reason upon the critical question of what an upright life is and must be. It is, therefore, a noble and important science.[2]

Norms of Human Acts

   a. **Law** – It is an ordinance of reason promulgated for the common good by one who has legitimate authority.
   b. **Conscience** – The practical judgment of reason upon individual acts as good to be performed or evil and avoided.

Importance Classes of Laws

   a. **Eternal Law** – It is God's eternal plan and providence for the universe. It is the divine reason or will which commands the preservation of the natural order of things and forbidding its disturbance.

b. **Natural Law** – it is eternal law as known to humans through reason. It is nothing than the participation of the rational creature in the eternal law of God and human comes to the knowledge of this law by the natural light of their reason.[3]

Properties of Natural Law

a. Universality – the natural moral law binds every person at all times and in all phases, or its basis is the very nature of humans.

b. Immutability – as soon as humans can use their reason, certain fundamental norms will become self-evident to humans.

c. Indispensability – no one is dispensed or excused in the observance of the natural law.

Types Of Natural Law As Presented Or Forbid As An Act

1. **Affirmative** – Laws which bind always, but not at the very moment. It states that human is morally obliged to adopt all ordinary means of preserving health and life.

2. **Negative** – Prohibitory laws. Deliberately willed as a means of destroying the health of life.

3. **Human Positive Law** – Law enacted by the church or state.

Professional Ethics – It is a branch of moral science that treats the obligations that a profession's members owe to the public, their profession, and their clients.[4]

Malpractice and Negligence

Malpractice – It involves any professional misconduct or any unreasonable lack of skill or fidelity in the performance of professional or fiduciary duties.

Profit Negligence – doing or failing to do that action which a reasonably prudent person would have done or would not have done in like or similar circumstances.

Elements of Negligence

1. Existence of Duty – there must be a moral obligation incumbent upon the person of doing or omitting something as mandated by his/her profession.
2. Failure to perform the duty – one fails to respond to the call of his/her profession.
3. Injury resulting from failure – there was grave harm resulting from not doing his/her duty or doing the wrong thing due to lack of knowledge.[5]

EXERCISES

Prepare in one clean bond paper

1. Define philosophy and trace its history

2. Explain the nature of man
3. Discuss the relationship of negligence and Malpractice to professional ethics.

Fill in the Blank

1. It comes from two Greek words. Its main objective is to seek the deepest explanation of existence and the nature of being.

   _____

2. _____wanted to call himself a person who just love wisdom or a "philosopher". One of the Greek thinkers.

3. Doctrine of Karl Marx

   _____

4. Doctrine of Immanuel Kant_____

5. Doctrine of Jean Paul Sarte

   _____

6. _____it is the awareness of sensation and the operation of external senses.

7. Latin work of Ethics

   _____

8. Greek of words _____

9. _____it tackles the basic principles in the life of man as a member of the society.

10. Deals with the basic principles which are the morality of human acts._____

11. Social observance required by good breeding

    _____

12. _____It is the branch of
    moral science that treats of the obligations which
    a member of a profession owes to the public, to
    his profession and to his clients.

13. _____is any technology
    using micro-organism or biological materials for
    technological purposes.

14. It is the eternal law as known to human through
    reason._____

15. Doing or failure to do that action which a
    reasonably prudent person would have done or
    would not have done in like or similar
    circumstances. _____

Chapter 4
Sanctity of Human Life

Scope:
    A – The principle of the sanctity of human life
    B – Man's Life: The duty of preserving it
    C – Analysis of commonly performed procedures

The Sanctity of Human Life – we view the sacredness of human life through a national or humanistic approach or by the religious or theistic approach.

Religious Approach – states that human life has dignity, and there is something sacred about it because it comes from God.

Rational/Humanistic Approach – these virtues that the experience of being alive generate the idea of sacredness, experiencing the elemental fear of its extinction and its sacredness is the most primordial of experience.

Two Levels of Moral Argumentation:

Moral Level – It's provided by the existing rules and norms of conduct that have been approved or validated before.

Ethical Level – It is in this sense that the sanctity of human life is an ethical principle. It declares that life is cherished, affirmed, respected, enhanced, and promoted.[1,2]

Man's Life

*All health workers who are facing different transitions in the delivery of health care services to the people have moved to a different level and the perception of their duty to preserve human life.

*Attruism** – in the changes and development of different ways of preserving people's lives through advanced technology, upscale services, and even the improvement of indigenous resources, health workers should be well guided by the principle that underlies these acts.

Law – is defined as an objective norm of morality in the ordinance of reason which dictates actions for the common good and promulgated by legitimate authority.

Kinds of Law

Eternal Divine Law – eternal plan of divine wisdom

Natural Divine Law – the participation of the rational being in the eternal plan of God

Positive Divine Law – a law that has been promulgated explicitly by GOD in the old and new testament.[3]

Human Law – has its immediate source of origin from human authority.

1. Civil Law – law made by the state
2. Canon Law – laws instituted by the church

Divine Law

1. Eternal law – is the divine reason on the wall of God commanding the preservation of the natural law and forbidding its disturbance.
2. Natural Law – is nothing other than the rational creature's participation in the eternal law of God and man comes to a knowledge of this law by the natural light of his reason.[2,3]

Properties of Natural Law

The universality of Natural Law – the natural moral law, binds every person at all times and in all places; its basis is the very nature of man.

Immutability of Natural Law – as soon as a man can use his reason, certain fundamental norms will become self-evident to man.

The indispensability of natural law – no one is dispensed or excused in the observance of the natural law.[4,5]

Scope and Application of Eternal Law

*Intrinsic and radial measure of our being. Only by observing that our actions be in agreement with our being and lead us to perfections.

*God gives us the strength to fulfill for eternity.

*Applies to every action of all creatures. It is an error to think that God does not ordain singular actions of beings.[6]

Eternal Law and Creatures

*Being may be subject to eternal law in two ways; through an internal moving principle or knowledge. Irrational creatures firstly follow the eternal law.

*Rational creatures follow eternal law in both ways. Like animals, they also have a natural inclination towards what is in agreement with the eternal law.

*Man can know what is good or bad but cannot decide what should be good or bad. Revelation teaches that the power to decide good and evil does not belong to man but God Alone.[6,7]

Properties of Natural Law

Universality – flows from human nature; it applies to all who share in nature. Implies that the rights and duties establishes apply to all men by the mere fact of being human. Its obligation is independent of culture, beliefs, environment, or circumstances; it stems from human nature, which all men equally possess because they are men.

Immutability – As long as their nature continues to be human, it flows from the immutability of human nature, which remains substantially the same at all times. The passage of time has led to new forms of human organization, changes in human relations, and general to different cultural orientations.[8]

Contents and Knowledge of Natural Law

*The obligation to love God above all creatures, together with the character proper to each creature, determines the right way to love all others good that is the content of natural law.

*The divine and natural law shows man how to follow is to practice the good and attain his end. The natural law states the first and essential precepts that govern the moral life.

*Natural law includes all the norms of conduct and only those that necessarily derive from human nature.[7]

Group O Propositions By S.T. Thomas and others

The first principle – one starting point of practical reasoning is that good is to be done and pursued, and evil is to be avoided. This directs human persons to the goods that fulfill them. These human goods do not have a moral value as such one chooses to establish them in immoral ways.

*He distinguishes various sorts of basic human goods, corresponding to "Natural Inclinations" of the human person not being exhaustive but rather illustrative.

Three Classifications of Inclinations:
1. Self-Preservation: It is common to all beings.
2. Animal Inclinations: It constitutes attributes such as mating and bringing up the offspring.
3. Goods according to nature of reason: These are specifically human inclinations, such as knowing the truth about God and living in society.

Three Categories Of Basic Goods Of Human Persons
1. Reflective or existential – human goods fulfill persons so far as they can make choices and are capable of good and evil.
    a. Self-integration or inner peace: It consists of harmony in one's judgments, feelings, and choices.
    b. Authenticity. It is the sincerity or harmony and consistency in one's judgments, feelings, choices, and behavior.
    c. Impersonal harmony. – It involves fraternity, friendship, and justice.
    d. Harmony with God – which is Religion
2. The three substantive human goods: wellbeing including health, integrity, a good that fills

human persons as physical beings, knowledge of the truth and appreciation of beauty that good fills human persons as intelligent beings and work, or skillful performance and activity that the person expands in the world, interact to it, transforms it, and finds fulfillment in doing so.

3. Marriage and family life are a component of humans [7,8]

The Immediate Conclusions or Secondary Principles

The purpose is to further specify the first moral principles by excluding immoral actions incompatible with a true integral human fulfillment.

Specific Moral Norms – this is made up of more specific moral norms which identify specific human actions that ought to be done or not done.[9]

Classification Of The Precepts Of Natural Law

1. Precepts from natural law – Which are found both in the old and new testaments. Example: Ten Commandments
2. Supernatural Precepts – man is destined for a supernatural end.

The Law of Charity – the bond of perfection is to love God in His intimate life, which is only possible through the supernatural strength of charity as God loves us, so we have to love others.

The Law of Perfect Freedom – since the new law is the love of charity, it is also the law of perfect freedom. Freedom is the tendency towards the good.

Grace Justification and Sanctity – the grace of God, has the power to justify us, that is, to cleanse us from our sins and to communicate to us.[6]

Remember: Whenever you perform actions that conform with the law, it is good. It guides you not only to become citizens who abide by certain rules but develop us to become moral individuals. The knowledge of the different aspects of laws will enable us to become more careful in these norms to help us fulfill our duty to preserve human life.

Exercise 2:

Prepare in one clean bond paper

1. Differentiate the religious from the rational approach in viewing the sacredness of life.
2. Explain and comprehend better the principle of sanctity of life.
3. Explain the nature of laws and identify their needs.

Chapter 5
Family and Marriage

A. Marriage: Basis of the Family

1. Marriage comes into existence when a man and a woman, forswearing all others, freely give themselves to one another through an act of irrevocable personal consent.[1]

2. At the heart of the act establishing marriage, there is a free, self-determining choice on the part of the man and the woman, through which they give themselves a new and lasting identity.

3. This man becomes this woman's husband, and she becomes his wife, and together they become spouses.

4. Marriage is established in and through the free, self-determining personal choice of the spouses; thus, it is a person-affirming reality.

The Sacredness of Sexuality[2]

4. Sexuality is a fundamental component of personality, one of its modes of being, manifestations, communicating to others, feeling, expressing, and living human love.

5. Feminity and Masculinity are complimentary gifts through which human sexuality becomes an integral part of the concrete capacity for love that God has inscribed in man and woman.[3]

6. Sexuality characterizes man and woman on the physical and psychological, and spiritual levels, making its mark on each of their expressions.

8. Conjugal love is an act of the total person and not an instinctive impulse; it embraces the totality of body and soul in the human person.[4]

9. The family is the necessary place where children are born and formed as the fruit of spouses' mutual love.

10. Marriage, on the other hand, is established by consent, and love is the object of that consent.

11. Consent generates a permanent bond which is the essence of marriage. Thus, love results in the marital institution.[5,6]

Characteristics of Human Love

1. It is human love both physically and spiritually.
2. It is total that a married person loves generously and shares a thing for undue reservation or selfish calculation.
3. It is faithful and exclusive
4. It is fruitful

The result of the spouses' total commitment is the child. This human person is a biological organism and a spiritual entity to a series of personal values.

Causes of Marriage

a. **Intrinsic Purpose** – the purpose of the action as Finis Operis
b. **Purpose of the agent** as Finis operantis

One thing is the actual intention of the spouses, and the other is the purpose or end of the institution itself of marriage.

1. **Final Cause** – (purpose of the institution).
2. **Efficient Cause** – the agent who brings it about
3. **Formal or constitutive cause** – what makes it a marriage
4. **Material Cause** – the living bodies of the spouses, over which they acquire mutual rights.[7]

The Blessings of Marriage

A man and woman give themselves the irrevocable identity of husband and wife and pledge to one another that they will honor and foster the "goods" or "blessings" of marriage.

Requirements Of Conjugal Love
    a. The good of the children
    b. The unity and indissoluble fidelity of marriage
    c. The good of the sacrament[8]

Can Marriage Go Wrong:
    a. The tendency to "divinize" human love, expecting from human love what any believers know only God can give.
    b. The tendency to confuse the purpose of marriage with the motive that leads individuals to marry.
    c. The tendency to see an opposition between these factors, instead of seeing them as complimentary to one another.

Family
Family is the Basic Unit of a society, the primary and natural school of life, the facilitator and the key to members total development, and the mini-domestic society wherein responsible citizens are formed, vested with rights and interests which must be served and defended by the state and the provider of the learning

environment for members to practice and learn values, heritage, friendship, and love.

A Community of Life and Love

Community – describes relationships among several persons. The birth of a child turns the conjugal communion naturally into a small community which is the family.

Privacy – which fosters individual autonomy and responsibility

Affection – which fosters sociability conducive to the development of the social virtues of a good citizen.[9]

Four General Tasks Of The Family
1. Forming a community of persons
2. Serving life
3. Participating in the development of society
4. Sharing in life and mission (spiritually)

Matrimony - has not been instituted by man. It is a natural institution authored by God. God made man essentially sociable. This sociability has its core of dividing the human race into two sexes: man and woman are attributed to each other and complement each other for procreation.

Essential properties of matrimony
1. **Unity** – the exclusive union of one man and one woman is clearly expressed.

    The most important consequence or moral dimension of unity is fidelity.

    The primary component of fidelity is LOVE because it motivates, impregnates, unifies, and dignifies the whole reality of matrimony.
2. **Indissolubility** – that matrimony is a state bond by its very reason of being is something that requires no demonstration.[10]

Exercise 3:

Prepare in one clean bond paper
1. Define Family and Marriage.
2. Explain the purpose and value of family

Sanctity of Human Life

Fill in the Blank

1. _____This states that human life has dignity and there is something sacred about it because of God.
2. _____
    3._____Two levels of Reasoning.
4._____ is defined as an objective norm of morality in ordinance of reason which dictates actions for the common good and promulgated by legitimate authority.

5. _____ An immediate source of origin from human authority.

6. _____ Is the divine reason on the will of God commanding the preservation of the natural law and forbidding its disturbance like sexual act.

7. _____ The capacity of using his reason, certain fundamental norms will become self-evident to man.

8. _____

9. _____ 10. _____

Classifications of Basic Inclinations.

11. _____ Refer to social organization.

12. _____ Refer to worship of God.

13. _____ The law expressly revealed by God.

14. _____ Human goods fulfil persons in so far as they are able to make choices and they are capable of moral good and evil.

15. _____ man is destined for a supernatural end.

Chapter 6
Foundation Of Conscience

Making moral decisions demands mature responsibility and seeks, understands reality, and is attentive to the wisdom of the past to discern the biases and demands of a particular situation. All of these efforts require a mature decision-maker. All of them hinge on the central issue of conscience.[1]

What is conscience?

It is "A little voice" inside our mind telling us what to do. It is the personal self. It tries to make a sound judgment about our basic moral questions.

It is the practical judgment of reason upon an individual act as good and to be performed or as evil and to be avoided.[2,3]

Before an action, conscience judges act as good and be performed or as evil and omitted. It is an immediate intellectual light shed upon the proposed action without which an act will not be called a human act.

33

After an action, conscience is a judgment of approval or disapproval. It is a moral judgment of what we have done.

Concepts of Conscience

1. **Heteronomous conscience** – tied to normative ethics, focussing solely on laws and obligations, commands and prohibitions, in such a way that there is hardly any place for the conscience to evaluate and decide.[4]

2. **Autonomous conscience** is subjective, ignoring the law and determining what is right and wrong.

Levels of Conscience

1. **Antecedent actual conscience** – the whole process of making a judgment in conscience before performing moral acts.

2. **Concomitant actual conscience** refers to our actual awareness of being morally responsible for the goodness or badness of a particular act we are carrying out.

3. **Consequent Actual Conscience** – involves the process of reflection on one's moral responsibility relative to past actions.[5,6]

Qualities of Conscience

1. **Personal Freedom**

    a. **Free** – one can assume a personal moral stand concerning a particular attitude or moral responsibility for a particular action in an unhindered or unimpeded way; to be able to claim full responsibility for a particular attitude or action.

    b. **Unfree** – one's moral attitude or responsibility for a particular action is hindered or impeded by obstacles or influences like force, fear, and anger.

2. **Objectives Values** are generally accepted as good because they conform to morality, for example, the divine reason that is eternally good and true.

    a. **Correct** – one's subjective perceptions, discernment, dictates, and decisions of conscience are in conformity with the objective moral values and demands that one strives to possess and express in one's actions.

    b. **Erroneous** – there is a lack of conformity between the objective values and the moral demands that they carry with them, subjective moral perceptions, discernment, dictates, and decisions that an individual has or makes in the habitual or actual levels of conscience.

c. **Culpable** – one is in error through one's fault and is therefore responsible for such an erroneous state of conscience.

d. **Inculpable** – one is in error through no fault of one's own, having erred in good faith while making reasonable attempts to form a correct conscience.

Vincible – can be corrected or overcome

Invincible – it is not possible to correct the error.

3.   **Moral Attitudes** -the process of making the transition from moral awareness to moral act.

a. **Lax** – Is remiss or careless in its efforts to perceive and internalize particular moral values.

b. **Strict** – when the conscience ends to judge moral obligations too harshly, especially in an excessively legalistic way, adhering more to the letter than the spirit of the law.

c. **Scrupulous** – a conscience that tends to judge sin to be present where there is none.

d. **Pharisaical** –tends to be self-righteous as for one's moral evaluation is concerned, while tending to be judgmental towards others, making unwarranted conclusions based on external observance of the law.

e. **Clear** – a conscience that confidently and freely acts and with due regard for perceiving, appreciating, and internalizing true values and making the proper transition in one's actual conscience when confronted with a moral decision regarding a particular way of acting.

f. **Callous** – this is the worst type of conscience because it has love sensitivity to sin and God as if it has no conscience.

4. Degree of Certitude

a. **Perplexed** – one judges it to be equally wrong to act in a particular way or refrain from acting, and therefore one cannot make a morally good choice.

b. **Doubtful** – the conscience, in its efforts to form a clear conscience on a particular attitude or way of acting, lacks sufficient evidence to make or leave judgment.

c. **Probable** – the conscience arrives at a point where it finds security in its formation of a moral attitude at the habitual level or of a practical judgment at the actual level, even while still admitting the possibility that the opposite may be true.

d. **Certain** – the conscience can reach a degree of certainty in its formation of moral judgment so that all practical doubts are resolved, and the new conscience is unhesitatingly clear in the actual process of making a sound discernment, dictate, and decision in the actual conscience.[7,8,9]

5. Responsible Conscience – free, correct, clear, and certain.

I. Dimensions of Conscience

a. General sense of value – are aware that we should do good and avoid evil. A sure sign of this general awareness is the fact that people argue about right and wrong. The desire to do the right thing reflects this general sense of value.

b. Search to discover the right course of action – probing into human behavior, and the world in the search for truth. If we are honest in our search, we turn to various sources for wisdom and guidance.

c. Actual Concrete Judgement – after searching for the truth, this is the point when a specific decision must be made.

II. Formation of Conscience – the conscience is the individual's Supreme Court, its judgment must be followed, but first, it must be formed into a fully mature and responsible conscience.

*Obey your conscience – this principle is true, but it should be properly understood. The dignity of the human person implies and demands the rectitude of the moral conscience or, in other words, one must try to make sure that one's moral judgment is right.

*Certain Conscience – the judgment about the goodness or evil of a particular action that is made without fear of being mistaken. Sins committed with a conscience that is both certain and erroneous are merely material sins. This would be the case of a person who does something wrong but is convinced that it is right.

Doubtful Conscience – is the suspension of the judgment on the moral goodness or evil of action because the intellect cannot see whether it is good or bad. It is due to natural causes, whether physical or moral, dealing with excessively strict persons, or even hidden pride.[10,11,12]

Two Types of Biased Conscience:

1. **Scrupulous conscience** – intellect with a tendency to scruples; decides that action is sinful based on weak or insufficient reasons.
   Symptoms: Excessive Anxiety; Fastidious and Obstinacy
2. **Lax conscience** – of the intellect with a tendency to laxity. Judges without sufficient reason that a certain action is not, or is only slightly, sinful.

> *Principles in resolving a doubtful conscience* – Strive to form a certain conscience before acting. This is done in various ways so that a practical certainty can be reached, which establishes a sufficient basis for acting in the amorally correct way.[13]

Two Types:

1. **Direct Solution of the Doubt** – this can be done by applying general principles to the particular case, consultation with experts, or employing references to other well-formed sources.

2. **Indirect Solution of the Doubt** – this may be done by having recourse to what is commonly called reflex principles, as expressed in certain prudence rules and various presumptions that establish a sufficient basis for resolving the practical doubt in such a way that one may then act with a clear conscience.[14]

> ***Principles used in moral discernment** – geared towards making correct moral decisions.

Two Types:

1. **The principle of Double-effect** – one act will have two different effects; one good and the other is bad. This principle helps us determine whether or not it is morally correct to perform one act, which will bring about good and evil effect.

2. **The principle of the lesser evil** – in conflicting situations where harm will result from either of two alternatives open to the agent, the rule of a person to choose the lesser evil.

3. **Principle of material and formal cooperation** – the one who cooperates somehow assists in the

4. carrying out of an immoral act, giving advice, providing necessary information, making necessary means available, or doing anything that makes the immoral act possible.

5. **Making Moral Decisions** – Choosing the action which does not fully promote humanity is not an easy task. Moral dilemmas confront us with profound complexity. A mature moral decision is not only a decision to do a good deed that "we ought to do" but also a choice made in good faith to make what we want ourselves "to be."[15]

Exercise 5
True or False

1. Gregor Mendel is an Australian Monk that discovered the laws of heredity.
2. It was determined that in the nuclei of the cells were thread-like strands called Mitochondrion.
3. Genetic engineering is the science that deals with the interaction of the genes in producing similarities and differences between individuals.
4. Scientist can't take useful genes from plant and animal cells.
5. Genetic testing is not used in detecting phenylketonuria.

6. Surrogacy is a biomedical technique whereby a fertilized ovum is implanted
    Into the uterus of another woman, who will carry a baby to term.
7. In case of embryo transfer, an ovum is removed from a woman's ovary by laparoscopy.
8. IVF involves conception outside the womb by artificial means.
9. Freezing and preservation of sperm at low temperature is called
    Cryopreservation.
10. Marital coitus should be timed as close as possible to the point of ovulation
    In the cycle.

Chapter 7

Transmission and Preservation of Life: The Case of Abortion and Contraception

Human life is sacred because, from the beginning, it involves the creative action of God, and it remains forever in a special relationship with the Creator.[1]

Abortion – the expulsions of a living fetus from the mother's womb before it is viable.

According to Dr. Andre E. Hellegers, "Abortion is defined as the termination of pregnancy, spontaneously or by induction, prior viability."[2]

Age of Viability – 20 weeks of gestation period wherein the fetus can survive in an extra-uterine environment.

Philippine Constitution, Article II, Section 12 of 1986 states, "The state recognizes the sanctity of life and shall protect and strengthen the family as a basic autonomous social institution. It shall equally protect the life of the mother and the life of the unborn from contraception".[3]

Types of Abortions:

Spontaneous abortion occurs naturally with no artificial means, which is usually lost in the first trimester. Genetics Findings:

a. Chromosomal structure and number are normal in both partners, but abnormal offspring can result sporadically and unpredictably.

b. One member of a couple is a carrier of a balanced translocation related to the abnormal development of the embryo or fetus. The abnormal development may be due to drugs or genetic makeup, faulty implantation due to abnormalities of the female generative tract, placental abnormalities, chronic maternal diseases, and endocrine imbalance.[4]

c. Most spontaneous abortion appears to be related to imperfections in sperm or ova or effects of teratogenic drugs.

d. Endocrine imbalance, particularly a reduction in progesterone and estrogen in early pregnancy, can retard the normal growth of the endometrial lining of the uterus.[5]

Classifications of Spontaneous Abortion

1. Threatened Abortion – the fetus is jeopardized by unexplained bleeding, cramping, and backache. The cervix is closed.

2. **Imminent Abortion** – Bleeding and cramping increase. The cervix dilates, membranes may rupture.

3. **Complete Abortion** – All products of conception are expelled. The cervix is dilated.

4. **Incomplete Abortion** – part of the products of conception are expelled. The cervix is a little open with one finger can admit.[6]

5. **Missed abortion** – the fetus dies in utero but is not expelled. Cervix is closed.

6. **Habitual Abortion** – Abortion occurs consecutively in three or more pregnancies.

Induced abortion – occurring as a result of the artificial or mechanical interruption. The first case is to get rid of the baby. The second case is for therapeutic purposes. Inducing a baby is intrinsically evil and qualified to homicide.

Moral and Ethical Point of View

*The direct and voluntary killing of an innocent human being is always gravely immoral, even when it is performed as a means to a good end. All wrong reasons violate the basic principle of any view on human life.[3]

Respect for the person and scientific research

*Research for experimentation on a human being cannot legitimize acts that are in themselves contrary to the dignity of a person or a moral law.

Respect for Health

*Life and physical health are precious gifts entrusted to us by God. We must take reasonable care of them, taking into account the needs of the other and the common good.

Respect for Bodily Integrity

*When performed for strictly therapeutic medical reasons.[7]

Effects of Abortion

Physically: Habitual Miscarriage, ectopic pregnancies, menstrual disturbances, and weight loss.

Psychologically: Guilt, suicidal tendencies, loss of sense of fulfillment, hostility, and anger

Abortion Under the Law

Legislative – laws that permit abortion with a maximum time limit. This states that abortion is possible up to a certain stage during pregnancy and is essentially at the women's request.

A law that allows abortion only for medical purposes

*Abortion is illegal in practice; Article III, Section 12 of the 1986 Constitution provides, "The state recognizes the sanctity of life and shall protect and strengthen the family as a basic autonomous social institution. It shall equally protect the life of the mother and the life of the unborn from conception."[2,3]

Ethics – the task of law is to protect the right of human beings, especially the most basic rights, and even more particularly, the rights of the most defenseless individuals.

Contraception – it is defined as the voluntary prevention of conception by the positive use of artificial means, which hinders the generative cells from uniting during the sexual act.

Methods of Contraception

1. **Folk Methods**

    Pre-coital/post-coital douche – vinegar and brine, which are highly spermicidal substances, are prescribed as pre-coital douche. Still, some people experience a burning sensation in the sensitive membranes of the genitals. This is believed to wash out sperms.

    Prolonged Lactation – it is believed that the prolongation of milk secretion or production in the mother's mammary glands could delay ovulation due to the hormonal imbalance occurring inside the mother's body.

    Withdrawal is withdrawing the penis from the vagina immediately before ejaculation and making ejaculation outside the vagina.[8]

    Coitus Reservatus – the male, withhold ejaculation just before orgasm and allows the erection to subside gradually; hence coitus is reserved.

    - This practice may lead to congestion of the prostate gland and seminal ducts, which could later create some physical and mental complications. Sex is the most intimate expression of love to his/her beloved partner and always a fulfilling and satisfying moment as a married couple.[9]

2. **Mechanical Methods** – this is the blocking of the sperm from entering the uterine cavity to prevent conception.

   Condom is a sheath latex rubber that the penis is inserted into before coitus to prevent the sperm from spilling out into the uterine cavity.

   Diaphragm – a dome-shaped latex rubber membrane place in the vagina to close the opening of the cervix to prevent entrance of the sperm. It is also called the cervical cap.

   Sponge – this is another variation of the diaphragm. It is rectangular with a string attached for easy removal.[10]

3. **Chemical Methods** – use spermicides that prevent conception by killing the sperm cells before entering the uterine cavity or reaching the fallopian tubes.

   Vaginal Suppositories – a small bullet-shaped substance similar to paraffin or a piece of candle that contains chemical capable of killing sperms.

   Vaginal Tablets – tablet, when moistened with water, is then inserted into the vagina 10-15 minutes before coitus. It melts at body temperature and forms a coat of foam to prevent sperm from entering the uterine cavity.

Vaginal Jellies, creams, and foams – are also inserted into the vagina shortly before copulation, immobilizing and killing the sperms. These spermicides are adequate for an hour.[11]

4. **Hormonal Methods**

   Contraceptive Pills – the pill is a combination of synthetic hormones, usually estrogen and progesterone. It helps maintain a constantly high hormonal level that prevents the ovary from releasing an egg; thus, conception will not occur, no matter how often the couple will engage themselves in sexual relations.

   Injections and Implants – a biodegradable pill implant, which is one centimeter long and can be injected through a large-bore needle, right through the woman's skin. This is the combination of cholesterol and hormones, which works for up to 3 years and does not require surgery for insertion.

5. **Abortifacients** – anything that cause abortion and expulsion of the fetus.

   Intrauterine Device is a small object made of plastic or stainless steel and comes in various shapes and sizes. This is placed or inserted inside the uterine cavity. Pregnancy is discontinued as it irritates and inflames the uterus lining so that the developing fetus that descends from the fallopian tube after it has been fertilized cannot implant itself in the uterus and eventually dies.[12]

DES (Diethystilbestrol) – known as a morning-after pill. It is a very strong kind of hormone that forces the endometrium or uterine lining to shed.

Prostaglandin – a powerful drug, taken or injected that causes violent contraction of the uterus that can expel out the product of conception; the fetus then could be expelled out either dead or alive.

Anti-pregnancy vaccine – this vaccine produces antibodies on the women that neutralize HCG. If the HCG level drops, then the woman menstruates, and a miscarriage occurs.

Low-dose type of contraceptive pills – this makes the endometrium not sufficiently prepared for implantation. This is related to the damage of the endometrium; hence miscarriage occurs. [10,12]

Exercise 7:

Fill in the blank:

1. _____ uses vinegar and brine which are highly spermicidal substances are prescribed as pre-coital douche but some people experiences a burning sensation in the sensitive membranes of the genitals. This is believed to wash out sperms.

2. _____it is belived that the prolongation of milk secretion or production in the mother's mammary glands could delay ovulation as a result of the hormonal imbalance occurring inside the mother's body.

3. _____this is withdrawing the penis from the vagina immediately before ejaculation and makes ejaculation outside the vagina.

4. _____the male withhold ejaculation just before orgasm and allows the erection to subside gradually, hence coitus is reserved.

5. _____ is the expulsions of a living fetus from the mother's wpomb before it is viable.

6. _____ is the 20 weeks of gestation period wherein the fetus can survive in an extra-uterine environment.

7. _____The state recognizes the sanctity of life and shall protect and strengthen the family as a basic autonomous social institution. It shall equally protect the life of the mother and the life of the unborn from contraception.

8. _____occurring naturally with no artificial means and this usually is lost in the first trimester.

9. _____ the fetus is jeopardized by unexplained bleeding, cramping and backache. The cervix is closed.

10. _____ Bleeding and cramping increase. The cervix dilates, membranes may rupture.

11. _____ All products of conception are expelled. The cervix is dilated.

12. _____the pill is a combination of synthetic hormones, usually estrogen and progesterone. It helps maintain a constantly high hormonal level which prevents the ovary from releasing an egg, thus conception will not take place, no matter how often the couple will engage themselves in sexual relations.

13. _____a biodegrable pill implant, which is one centimetre long and can be injected through a large-bone needle, right

through woman's skin. This is the combination of cholesterol and hormones, which works up to 3 years and does not require surgery for insertion.

14. _____ anything that cause abortion and expulsion of the fetus.

15. _____ this is a small object made of plastic or stainless steel and comes in various shapes and sizes. This is place or inserted inside the uterine cavity. Pregnancy is discontinued as it irritates and inflames the lining of the uterus in such a way that the developing fetus that descends from the fallopian tube, after it has been fertilized, cannot implant itself in the uterus and eventually dies.

Chapter 8
Family Planning and Sterilization: Methods and Moral Responsibility

Planning a family is an inevitable moral responsibility. One of the basic, highly intimate, and important parts of human life is producing sensible, reasonable decisions in a climate of freedom and love.

God has created human beings not only on His collaborators in building the world but also as free, responsible agents.

This area of life falls under the heading of free human beings, action used to be characterized by a clear sense of responsibility, and there is no reason why human reproduction should not be one of them.[1]

Moral Lesson of Student Nurse is:

1. Value the importance and inevitability of family planning and sterilization

2. Analyze the different methods of family planning and sterilization
3. Decide on a morally effective and responsible means.
4. Able to give responsible justification when faced in a situation that involves family planning and sterilization issues in any setting that you are working
5. Be responsible parents in the future and help others build up their families as responsible parents committed to using a morally acceptable method.[2]

The World Health Organization defines Family Planning as a way of thinking and living that is adapted voluntarily upon the basis of knowledge, attitudes, and responsible attitudes and decisions by individuals and couples to promote the health and welfare of the family group (WHO,1971).[3]

Nurses are task to perform:

1. Forming a community of persons
2. Serving Life
3. Participating in the development of society
4. Sharing in the life and mission of our faith.
   The integral Family Planning must therefore concern itself and consider the health and welfare of the individual member so that

they will be able to carry out individually the mission and perform their task as family.

Methods of Family Planning Or Birth Control

1. **Natural or Behavioral Methods** – they are the natural means that couples can avail themselves so that conception will not occur.

a. **Rhythm or Calendar Method** – this method is also known as Basal Body Temperature Method. This is used to indicate the time of ovulation. To avoid conception, the couple should abstain from sexual relations when a sudden rise of body temperature occurs and is sustained for about three days.[4]

b. **Ovulation Method or Billing Method** – this technique is based on the mucus discharge from the vagina as a sign of impending ovulation, which signals the beginning of the unsafe period.[5]

c. **Sympto-thermal method** is a combination of the temperature method and the mucus method with pain symptoms in cervical charges.

2. **Artificial and Natural Family Planning** – can strictly be identified with contraception. It is the decision to use unnatural contraceptive methods to plan the size of the family or the number of

children they will beget or as a means for spacing children.

3. **Sterilization** – is a medical or surgical intervention that is performed in the patient, man or woman, incapacity for generation, whether organic or functional, temporary or permanent.

   a. **Therapeutic sterilization** – which is inevitably required by and for the health or survival of the person. The principle rules it, for the sexual organs are, like other bodily organs, integrating parts which must yield to the good of the whole.[6]

   b. **Direct sterilization** – regardless of the ostensible benefits and justification in the light of which it is presented-will always be a grave violation of natural law. It is a gross abuse of man's right over his faculties, which God has given him to be employed in the scope of their natural purposes.

Types of Sterilization
1. Euphonic – in the interest of conserving the voice.
2. Ascetic – designed to conquer the sin of lust.
3. Punitive –to punish crimes.

4. Eugenic – seeking to avoid the transmission of hereditary defects.

5. Hedonistic –to evade the complications and responsibilities of procreation without giving up the sexual pleasure.

6. Demographic –to control the birthrate through implementing its population policy.

7. Preventive – to render impossible pregnancies that might aggravate sickness that already exist without any causal relation with the sexual function.

Methods of Sterilization

1. **Tubal Sterilization** – Salpingectomy; consists of the ligation or electrocoagulation of both fallopian tubes. It is highly an effective contraceptive method. It is usually irreversible, although there are techniques of recanalization.

2. **Vasectomy** – in males refers to bilateral ligation of vas deferens which impedes the passage of spermatocytes.[7]

Pain, Analgesia and Euthanasia

In the health care service that we are in, the demand for assistance to have one's life ended should be heard. As such, it is greatly hoped that one presents a moral stand.

Pain – is a complex, abstract, personal experience. It is an unpleasant sensation caused by noxious stimulation of the sensory nerve endings.

Types of Pain
1. **Acute pain** – is intense and of short duration; it follows acute injury, disease, or type of surgery and has a rapid onset.
2. **Chronic pain** – generally characterized by pain lasting longer than six (6) months. The pain can be continuous or intermittent and can be as intense as acute pain.[8]

Behavioral Characteristics of Pain
1. Is self-protective; guards the painful area places hands over the area.
2. Has narrowed focus; cannot think of anything but the pain, has reduced attention span.
3. Withdraws from social contact avoids conversation or social contacts.
4. Has impaired thought process
5. Demonstrates distraction behavior, including moaning, rocking, crying, restlessness, or seeking out other people or activities.

Analgesic – Method of Pain relief.
   a. There are cases in which it is a grave obligation to accept physical pain.
   b. There is no general obligation to seek or accept physical pain.

c. Analgesic is, therefore, in itselfliclit.

d. There are cases in which analgesia could be obligatory.

e. There are cases in which analgesia could be obligatory.

Syndrome – is considered the final phase of many progressive chronic diseases when all available treatment has been exhausted, and the vital level of irreversibility has been reached.

Death – is more complicated than it used to be; it is a time of ethical conflict.

Euthanasia – derives from the Greek word eu (good) and thanatos (death). It etymologically signifies good death, a pleasant, gentle death without awful suffering. It may be defined as an action or omission, that by its very nature, or intention, causes death to eliminate pain.[9]

Kinds of Euthanasia

1. **Suicidal Euthanasia** – when the subject himself a love or with the help of the others resorts to lethal means to interrupt or suppress his life. Therefore, it is done with the subject's consent.

2. **Homicidal Euthanasia**
   a. **Piety** – is performed to liberate a person from a terrible disease, severe senility.
   b. Social or Eugenic – seeks to eliminate lives devoid of vital value or to purify the race.

3. **Ortothanasia** – means normal death. The subject is left to die by omitting any medical assistance—death in due time considered ethical.[9]

4. **Positive or Negative** – positive provokes death through adequate intervention. Negative is the result of omitting necessary medical support.

5. **Active and Indirect** – there is a growing tendency today to impose the terminology. Seeks to alleviate a patient of his sufferings with the accompanying risk of shortening his life.

6. **Painless Death** – drugs to modify or suppress pain or not to provoke death.

Chapter 9
The Right to Life

Man has useful or indirect ownership of his own body, but not an absolute privilege. God gave us life, and only God has the right to take that life back. Therefore, it is vital to know and understand some legal and moral implications over an individual's bodily integrity.[1]

Life is the result of the harmonious functioning of a series of organs. However, a diseased organ can threaten the entire human body at a certain moment. The problem then arises as to whether or not the organ should be extirpated or eliminated. This is the term "mutilation."

Principle of Totality – is the basis of mutilation. In as much as they are parts, the parts of a physical whole are ordained to the good of the whole. The reason is that this is good, which gives fundamental meaning to the whole. It is applied to the body, that some part or function becomes a threat to the whole body.

Health workers have legal and ethical responsibilities to understand the underlying causes and management of improperly using drugs. When caring for substance abuse patients, they must be aware of their values and possess a positive and caring attitude. Otherwise, they cannot develop a therapeutic relationship with clients if personal values interfere with acceptance and understanding of their needs.

Crisis intervention is necessary for acute and repeated episodes of suicidal tendencies. Professionals should be alert for warning signs or signals of destructive behavior to instigate prompt intervention.

Suicide is always a most grievous sin or offense, and usually, there is no time to repent and ask for forgiveness. This act violates charity towards oneself and justice towards God and society.[2]

The Virtue of Justice

There are no small parts to play when it comes to the career of being a health care provider. Each of us has been carefully crafted, intricately designed by God, to fulfill what He views as a crucial call in the big picture of this thing we call life.[3]

A person is guided by the choices he makes. A life full of morally good choices makes an integrally good person, a person with good character, the different aspects of a person's good character are called virtues.

A natural virtue can be defined as a "good habit of the mind which always inclines to do well."[4]

Two Classifications of Natural Virtue

Intellectual virtue – produce specific inclinations in the human intellect in relation to the knowledge of the truth.

   a. **Understanding** – the inclination to know the first intellectual principles clearly and intimately.

   b. **Science** – the inclination to relate effects to causes and to deduce from know principles.

   c. **Wisdom** – the inclination to consider every object known in relation to its most profound cause.[5]

   d. **Prudence** – the inclination to pronounce the right judgment on the proper human behavior. This virtue affects the will.

   e. **Art or technique** – the inclination to find the best way to perform specific human actions, like playing the piano, carving a statue, tuning up a car, or making a logical conclusion.

Moral Virtues – refer to human behavior and are in themselves morally good. This is inclinations of human faculties towards the right behavior in what refers to the means to reach the objective.[6,7]

Justice – a moral standard of all men to one another, requiring them to perform their social and moral and legal obligations to each other. In this meaning, it is synonymous with equity in its largest sense.

Ethics are a fundamental part of nursing. All nurses should have respect for their patients, protect their rights and maintain dignity. Nurses should create a favorable environment for mutual trust and respect between the patients and rest of healthcare professionals.[5,8]

NOTES

CHAPTER 1

1. "Tisdale's Topics." Jackson Advocate, vol. 77, no. 48, Jackson Advocate, 3 Sept. 2015, p. 4A.
2. nursingblog: Management of 'Nursing Shortage' based on https://nursingblogging.blogspot.com/2010/01/among-many-nursing-roles-leadership-and.html

CHAPTER 2

1. IT - Engineering. https://sites.google.com/education.nsw.gov.au/qhssubjectselection-stage5/tas-and-art-faculty/it-engineering
2. Learning Objectives - Eberly Center - Carnegie Mellon .... https://www.cmu.edu/teaching/designteach/design/learningobjectives.html
3. Bioethics | Bioethics | Natural Law - Scribd. https://www.scribd.com/doc/17731601/Bioethics
4. Chapter 1-nature Of Philosophy [ylyxzkpjgvnm]. https://idoc.pub/documents/chapter-1-nature-of-philosophy-ylyxzkpjgvnm
5. Morality, Ethics, and the Death Penalty Example | Graduateway. https://graduateway.com/morality-ethics-and-the-death-penalty/

CHAPTER 3

1. ETHICS, PROFESSIONAL CONDUCT, AND THE REAL ESTATE LAW.

https://www.assess.biz/exams/file_download.asp?file=ETHICS.pdf

2. Bioethics | Bioethics | Natural Law - Scribd. https://www.scribd.com/doc/17731601/Bioethics

3. Chapter 1-nature Of Philosophy [ylyxzkpjgvnm]. https://idoc.pub/documents/chapter-1-nature-of-philosophy-ylyxzkpjgvnm

4. https://books.openedition.org/obp/4422?lang=en #:~:text=Aquinas's%20Natural%20Law%20Theory%20contains,we'd%20better%20start%20there%E2%80%A6

5. https://iep.utm.edu/natlaw/

CHAPTER 4

1. https://www.ncbi.nlm.nih.gov/pmc/articles/PMC2043345/

2. https://www.jstor.org/stable/797022

3. http://press.georgetown.edu/book/georgetown/sanctity-human-life

4. https://www.cmalliance.org/about/beliefs/perspectives/sanctity-of-life

5. https://cbhd.org/content/sanctity-life

6. https://cbhd.org/content/sanctity-life

7. Library : Compendium of the Social Doctrine of the Church .... https://www.catholicculture.org/culture/library/view.cfm?recnum=7213

8.] is for val ed :)). https://www.slideshare.net/heartplusbrain/is-for-val-ed

9. PPT - God the Lawgiver PowerPoint Presentation, free .... https://www.slideserve.com/orsen/god-the-lawgiver

CHAPTER 5

1. 29. Marriage, the Origin of the Family - Faith Seeking https://fsubelmonte.weebly.com/29-marriage-the-origin-of-the-family.html

2. https://www.yourarticlelibrary.com/sociology/ki
   nship-and-family/3-forms-of-family-on-the-basis-
   of-structure-and-marriage/31303
3. https://opentextbc.ca/introductiontosociology2nde
   dition/chapter/chapter-14-marriage-and-family/
4. https://www.princeton.edu/~anscombe/position_
   statements/Family%20and%20Marriage.htm
5. https://www.ncbi.nlm.nih.gov/books/NBK310966
   /
6. https://perspectives.pressbooks.com/chapter/fami
   ly-and-marriage/
7. https://www.ncbi.nlm.nih.gov/pmc/articles/PMC
   4012696/#:~:text=The%20most%20commonly%20re
   ported%20major,blamed%20themselves%20for%20t
   he%20divorce.
8. https://www.jstor.org/stable/352597
9. https://www.verywellmind.com/common-
   marriage-problems-and-solutions-3144958
10. https://bestlegalchoices.com/6-common-causes-of-
    marital-problems/

CHAPTER 6

1. National University of Singapore Personal
   Statement .... https://phdessay.com/national-
   university-of-singapore-personal-statement/
2. There was one drug that the doctors thought might
   save her ....
   https://www.coursehero.com/file/p7dbf278/Ther
   e-was-one-drug-that-the-doctors-thought-might-
   save-her-It-was-a-form-of/
3. Essay on Conscience - 537 Words - StudyMode.
   https://www.studymode.com/essays/Conscience-
   1367391.html
4. 5. Conscience - Faith Seeking Understanding.
   https://fsubelmonte.weebly.com/5-
   conscience.html
5. https://courses.lumenlearning.com/boundless-
   psychology/chapter/introduction-to-
   consciousness/#:~:text=of%20psychoanalytic%20th
   eory.-

,Freud%20divided%20human%20consciousness%20
into%20three%20levels%20of%20awareness%3A%2
0the,id%2C%20ego%2C%20and%20superego.

6. https://www.barrettacademy.com/levels-of-
    consciousness
7. https://plato.stanford.edu/entries/conscience/#:~:
    text=On%20any%20of%20these%20accounts,us%20(
    as%20opposed%20to%20external
8. https://www.lilleoru.ee/en/art-of-conscious-
    change-conscious-person-seven-qualities
9. https://www.ncbi.nlm.nih.gov/pmc/articles/PMC
    3956087/
10. https://philosophyterms.com/conscience/
11. https://www.consciencelaws.org/religion/religion
    040.aspx#:~:text=II.,The%20Formation%20of%20Co
    nscience&text=This%20never%2Dending%20search
    %20which,%22formation%22%20of%20his%20consc
    ience.
12. https://www.archspm.org/faith-and-
    discipleship/catholic-faith/what-does-it-mean-to-
    have-a-well-formed-conscience/
13. https://libraryguides.saic.edu/learn_unlearn/foun
    dations6#:~:text=Conscious%20Bias%3A%20Biased
    %20attitudes%20about,action%20more%20than%20
    conscious%20biases.
14. https://nccc.georgetown.edu/bias/module-
    3/1.php
15. National University of Singapore Personal
    Statement .... https://phdessay.com/national-
    university-of-singapore-personal-statement/

CHAPTER 6

1. Diversity & Dignity - University of Dallas.
    https://udallas.edu/diversity-dignity/index.php
2. nursing kingdom: September 2009.
    https://uznursingkingdom.blogspot.com/2009/09
    /
3. "Philippines : Solons Want Media Outlets Airing or
    Publishing Positive Advocacies given Tax

Incentives." MENA Report, Albawaba (London) Ltd., May 2014, p. n/a.

4. German Incest Case – Aardvarchaeology – by Dr. Martin https://aardvarchaeology.wordpress.com/2008/03/14/german-incest-case/
5. Which drugs help regulate the growth of the endometrial https://e-eduanswers.com/medicine/question513781166
6. Unit 7 - Complications of Pregnancy with pictures, revised https://www.coursehero.com/file/20705256/Unit-7-Complications-of-Pregnancy-with-pictures-revised-1/
7. Catechism of the Catholic Church - Paragraph # 2288. http://www.scborromeo.org/ccc/para/2288.htm
8. Counseling/Educational Information: Coitus Interruptus https://www.mfhs.org/wp-content/uploads/2014/12/Counseling-Educational-Information-Coitus-Interruptus-Withdrawal.pdf
9. YOU HAVE TO TRY BEFORE YOU BUY — Sabrina Peters. https://sabrinapeters.com/youhavetotrybeforeyoubuy/you-have-to-try-before-you-buy
10. https://www.nhs.uk/conditions/contraception/what-is-contraception/
11. https://www.familyplanning.org.nz/advice/contraception/contraception-methods
12. https://www.cdc.gov/reproductivehealth/contraception/index.htm

CHAPTER 8

1. A study to assess the knowledge, practice and attitude on https://1library.net/document/zpn03n4y-knowledge-practice-attitude-temporary-permanent-contraceptive-selected-coimbatore.html

2. Males non-compliance driving Anambra's low Contraceptives .... https://www.thenews-chronicle.com/males-non-compliance-driving-anambras-l-ow-contraceptives-prevalence-rate-expert/
3. How Family Planning Can Benefit You: Women's Clinic of the .... https://www.wcrgv.com/blog/how-family-planning-can-benefit-you
4. Womens' Health. https://melanieshealth.blogspot.com/
5. Ethics-Family Planning and Sterilization & Abortion https://www.coursehero.com/file/28046821/Ethics-Family-Planning-and-Sterilization-Abortion-MIDTERMdocx/
6. Movie Review - Ebola: The Plague Fighters (1996). https://www.ttu.edu/biodefense/reviews/ebola.pdf
7. Faith Seeking Understanding (vol. 2). https://where-you-are.net/ebooks/faith-seeking-understanding-v2-charles-belmonte.docx
8. HESI review - ACUTE AND CHRONIC PAIN Acute pain is intense https://www.coursehero.com/file/36722955/HESI-reviewdocx/
9. nursing kingdom: September 2009. https://uznursingkingdom.blogspot.com/2009/09/

CHAPTER 9

1. Mark Todd Shot Fort Hood Suspect - hiphopmusic.com. http://www.hiphopmusic.com/best_of_youtube/2009/11/mark_todd_shot_fort_hood_suspect.html
2. nursing kingdom: September 2009. https://uznursingkingdom.blogspot.com/2009/09/

3. Training for the Gold (Arousal Control) – Dream. https://teneishajohnsondream.wordpress.com/2019/02/11/training-for-the-gold-arousal-control-2/
4. Faith Seeking Understanding (vol. 2). https://where-you-are.net/ebooks/faith-seeking-understanding-v2-charles-belmonte.docx
5. Importance of Ethics in Nursing. https://www.nursingwritingservices.com/blog/393-importance-of-ethics-in-nursing
6. Ashcroft, Richard E., Dawson, Angus, Draper, Heather, and McMillan, John R. (2006). **Principles of Health Care Ethics**.
7. Guido, Ginny Wacker (2001). **Legal and Ethical Issues in Nursing Third Edition**. Prentice-Hall, Inc, Upper Saddle River, New Jersey
8. Myers, David and Jeeves, Malcom (2003). **Psychology Through the Eyes of Faith**. Council for Christian Colleges & Universities, HarperCollins Publishers, New York.

www.ingramcontent.com/pod-product-compliance
Lightning Source LLC
Chambersburg PA
CBHW072233170526
45158CB00002BA/881

*9 7 8 1 1 0 5 7 7 1 4 1 5 *